LIVING A SPIRITUAL LIFE™

Ground your divine essence here on earth.

Discover what spirituality means to you, by consciously
living between the two worlds of the sacred and the mundane.

LIVING A SPIRITUAL LIFE COPYRIGHT

Please note:

The written or spoken information, ideas, procedures and suggestions contained and presented in 'LIVING A SPIRITUAL LIFE' workshops and books are meant for educational purposes only and is not for diagnosis. It should not be used as substitute for your physician's advice. 'LIVING A SPIRITUAL LIFE' is not therapy and is not intended to replace the recommendations of a licensed health practitioner. It is the responsibility of the reader to consult with their own medical Doctor, Counselor, Therapist or other competent professional regarding any condition before adopting any of the suggestions in this book.

LIVING A SPIRITUAL LIFE™

Dedicated to awakening the Sacred
which inherently lies within us
and to receiving the Blessings
and Grace of these Divine forces.

MISSION STATEMENT

To guide and facilitate women
in becoming their most beautiful and radiant selves.

To acknowledge and embrace the well of love
and power which lies within all women and to ignite the
awakening and embodying of this life force.

To empower each woman, through exquisite self-care and love,
to live her fullest life possible, and to walk her path of wisdom
and truth, as she shares this light and knowledge
with all beings.

IN DEEP GRATITUDE

Thank you

The creation, birth and life of 'A Woman's Truth' would not have been possible without the love, support and devotion from the following angels in my life:

My beautiful daughter Megan who naturally embodies the teachings of living in her truth and integrity, thank you for the creative gift of the beautiful artwork. Helena Nelson-Reed for her generosity of spirit in allowing her extraordinary artwork, which embodies the teachings so magnificently, to grace the covers. Dennise Marie Keller for her unwavering support and dedication to the teachings and for proofing, editing, aligning and translating my vision into the technical world of manifestation. Dan Fowler for his creative genius and dedication. Lucy Alexander and Suzanne Ryan, my dearest friends for their amazing editing and wholehearted encouragement. Monica Marsh for her commitment, support and belief in the workshops. Maggie Crawford, my mum, for her proofing and for being a living example of the teachings. Cait Myer and Katie Steen for their patience and ability to decipher my handwriting and for formatting the books. Bethany Kelly for her support. Deborah Waring for holding the space for the conception of 'A Woman's Truth' to be born and for her insight in the first year of teaching and Emmanuel for believing in my vision.

My mentors and teachers Rod Stryker, Adyashanti and Alison Armstrong, Max Simon and Jeffrey Van Dyk for their continuous and guiding light in my life, their never-ending belief in my potential and for always teaching me the way to evolve into my highest and most potent self. And to all of you beautiful and courageous women who are committing to living your truth and transforming into your most radiant selves,

thank you.

PRELUDE

An Overture to the Living A Spiritual Life.

Miranda Barrett is a rare and extraordinary writer, teacher and guide. Her years of guiding others, clarity and sensitivity allow her to transmit the essential wisdom of both modern science and ancient wisdom with great expertise and inspired elegance. Living a spiritual life is a treasure for those seeking lasting fulfillment and peace.

~ Rod Stryker
Pre-eminent yoga and meditation teacher,
author of best selling The Four Desires

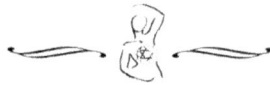

I will probably never forget meeting Miranda Barrett. It was almost a decade ago at a yoga workshop. She immediately stuck out to me. Not because of her beauty (which is apparent), nor her words (which have all the appeal of a sexy English lullaby), but for more subtle reasons.

She held something. Moreover, whatever it was that she was holding made something powerful radiate out from her milky skin and knowing gaze. She was raw and perfectly imperfect and vulnerable and wise all at once. She was also one of the rare women I have encountered who had the courage to give me hard advice in a loving way. It seems that Miranda gives us this book, *Living a Spiritual Life,* as a very personal "how-to" manual on how we can awaken the force of Love within ourselves. Perhaps that "something powerful" I saw in Miranda that day was just the result of the practices you now hold in your hand, made manifest in her.

I was lucky enough to be personally mentored by Miranda for a period following our meeting. She challenged me. She held me like a mother. She cursed. She emoted. In addition, she asked me to get real about difficult things like sex, money, food-addictions and power. However, there was one thing that Miranda said to me that has since stuck with me, embedding itself into my body like an imprint in hot wax: "Katie," she said, "a woman's *feminine* heart is her womb."

This book is an exploration on how a woman can reconnect to that sacred space of spirituality within her own body and her own life. Through these words and daily practices, you will find a reconnection to the *shakti* of your own feminine heart. *Shakti* can be defined as a living, powerful spiritual potential that lives in our body. It is begging to be awakened. Awakening our *shakti* requires a deep willingness to feel. It also requires a vulnerable surrender into what *is* -be it an emotion, a sensation or an intuition. It also requires, as Miranda demonstrates, a willingness to weave spiritual practices into the fabric of daily life.

For thousands of years, this spirit-infused energy has been repressed, feared and demonized - particularly in women. Miranda's book, *Living a Spiritual Life,* teaches us how to reclaim this feminine spirit-force as a gateway into the healing of our collective wounding. Her book is also an invitation to a re-engagement with the collective *shakti* of woman-kind. I see her and her work as one of many powerful female forces on this planet, working diligently to awaken the soul of women so that perhaps our world can be a better place for future generations.

I read this book like a ravenous tigress - quickly and with a voracious desire to know and possess. I then read it a second time like a receptive, watery mama, letting her words and time-tested lady-wisdom steep my flesh like much-longed-for nectar. Read it any way you please. Nevertheless, read it. I dare to give yourself the gifts of deep self-care, self-inquiry and most importantly, self-compassion. In this way, you will have no choice but to become a force of Love in the world. We need you.

With all my feminine heart,

~ Katie Silcox
Author of Healthy, Happy, Sexy - Body + Soul Balance
Through Ancient Ayurveda

LIVING A SPIRITUAL LIFE™

Gems of Consciousness

A DAILY PRACTICE
commit to Yourself

*F*ollow these simple steps daily as a way to instill and strengthen your heartfelt resolve to love yourself. This will help to keep you aligned, transforming and on track, giving you a stable foundation for the rest of your life. As a gift to yourself, please mark the teachings as you read them through and congratulate yourself with each one. See each day as a commitment to take exquisite care of yourself.

A LIFE WORTH LIVING

"Never give from your well.
Always give from your overflow."
~ Rumí

All too often as women, your own needs are denied for the benefit of others as you orchestrate your life through demands and expectations you feel responsible for. Unfortunately, this can leave you without the juice and energy needed to be present fully and to enjoy life. During these readings, you will continually discover more about who you truly are and learn the tools needed to live your most authentic and fulfilling life possible. From this place, you will experience being 'full to overflowing' and all the joy and energy this brings.

As you delve into these teachings, you will explore, laugh, study, share, and freely express who you are. In this sacred space, you will ultimately learn your truth as a woman in order to shine, to embody your own beauty, believe in your own worth, and take exquisite care of yourself. For only in this way can you truly be of service.

During these guidebooks, many of the basic needs of women will be explored such as sleep, nutrition, creativity, movement and time to replenish. A topic has been chosen for each book and a cohesive and practical foundation is laid out to inspire and guide you. This will bring about a new strength and resolve which will allow your needs to become a priority, without letting your outer world dictate otherwise. By the end of our time together, the concept of being confident, loving, serene and passionate will no longer be a distant fantasy. Instead, these and many other extraordinary qualities that you naturally embody as a woman will flow with ease, grace and love.

With life's demands so high, it has become imperative that your needs are first acknowledged, honored and then taken care of. From this vantage point, your relationship with yourself then has the potential to be transformed into one of self-love. The beauty is this in turn creates a life that not only fulfills you and your life's purpose, but also allows everyone touched by your presence to receive this gift.

I look forward to spending this precious time with you.

Welcome to A Woman's Truth.

Sincerely and with love,

Miranda

SPIRITUALITY

we are spiritual beings on a human journey.

Certain words seem to invoke the world of the mystical and divine. It can also be said that specific actions, choices or intentions allow a human being to embody and live in this unseen and revered realm of otherworldliness.

The words spirituality, mysticism and holiness call upon divine meaning and are related to matters of the sacred. They have a spiritual intent or reality that is neither apparent to the five senses nor obvious to the intellect. If their meaning is so intangible and unrelated to the realm of survival, why then is it important to spend precious time, money or energy seeking to imbue your essence with such a sanctified domain? It seems a person can certainly choose to live a good life with integrity and honor without having any connection to a spiritual practice.

"My father was a living example of this. He was an out and out atheist. He had no belief in God, a higher power or even that he would exist at all after his death. To his dying day, this did not change. Yet he certainly lived his life fully and was a good, decent, upright human being." ~ Miranda

What are the benefits for committing and carving out precious time to connect to an unseen world or to spend time in prayer, silence or meditation? What is being offered here is to give yourself the gift to freely choose what is right for you. In this context, spirituality does not necessarily have anything to do with God or religion. Both of these may be part of your spiritual practice, but for this particular journey, they are certainly not a necessity.

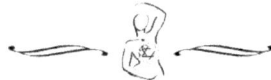

*"Life is full of relationships,
including the one with our own divinity."
~ Anonymous*

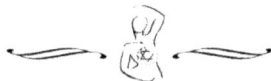

I

As a human, you seem to have a foot in two worlds. One is that of the physical, material and mundane world where you get to see, touch and feel your existence. In this realm, you identify with your physical body as being who you are. Moreover, with all its intelligence and brilliant design, this miracle of a body does an extraordinary job of carrying you through your life experience.

This premise of honoring the physical form has been the foundation in the teachings of 'A Woman's Truth'. The concepts of how to respect, take care of and nourish this precious temple that houses your being are highlighted and set in stone. Yet the trouble with focusing primarily on the physical form is that emotions such as fear, limitation and immortality can tend to arise and dominate your world.

when a body is born, the body itself will certainly die.

Think of all the advertising money and time spent attempting to defy death. Supplements, elixirs, surgeries, medications, spas, diets, are all used to cheat death. Yet it is often forgotten that to take care of the body on a daily basis is a relatively inexpensive ordeal as it is a natural, intuitive reaction based on your survival.

◆ 'I am tired' ~ therefore sleep.

◆ 'I am hungry' ~ then eat.

◆ 'I am getting burnt' ~ get out of the sun.

◆ 'I am thirsty' ~ so drink.

To take care of this amazing instrument of a body is not complicated. You all have tools that can certainly prolong life and hinder illness. Yet, no matter how you attempt to dodge the bullet, the ultimate ending still does occur. You will die.

This is where spirituality comes in.

Because the physical world is rather limited and mortal, it tends to connect you strongly to your ego, which is all about survival. Obviously, living to tell the tale is imperative. Yet, unfortunately, many of these survival instincts can become the bane of your existence. This includes emotions such as anger, greed, envy, jealousy, the belief that there is not enough to go around and the instinct of fight or flight.

These programs keep you in the lower level of your more animalistic instincts, therefore not allowing room for the higher realms of love, compassion or kindness. When you connect to the realm of spirituality or energy, you are placing a foot in the other camp. The concept of infinite, immortal and endless possibilities comes alive. Human beings are energy in a physical form.

This means your frequency has slowed down enough to become material. It seems one gift of being human is that you do have the ability to reside in both of these worlds, that of the material and the spiritual in the same moment. The aspect that connects to your spiritual Self has no fear of death. It knows you are energy that comes from an infinite source and that when the body dies, you ultimately return to this source. Whether you believe in reincarnation or not is immaterial. The point is to remember that the expression of you as a human being will die, yet you as a vehicle of energy are infinite and will always live on.

Unfortunately, as you go through daily life, the physically mundane world can often eclipse the magic and beauty of creation itself. When you choose to connect to spiritual practices, this ability to remember who you truly are, which is endless sources of energy, is kept alive. All of existence is a living embodiment of creation itself, a flower, a newborn baby or even a laptop.

*It is all about remembering
and making choices, which remind you of your eternal essence.*

For you to freely become the unique expression and reality of your spiritual essence, it is vital to keep in mind how patterns and many of your daily actions and habits were born before you. Beliefs and ways of being are passed down through your ancestors and family-line. Unless these attitudes are questioned, they can unconsciously become part of who you are as you live in the shadows of the past.

Religion, traditions and spiritual practices can certainly play a part in this role. Some of you may have rebelled against what you were taught, or embraced your religious upbringing. You may have chosen a new path or opted out completely. There is no judgment here. It is about finding your truth.

The question to ask yourself is:

◈ Are you still living in reaction to your parents, culture or upbringing, or is your spirituality a decision made from your own authentic truth?

As you embark on this journey of discovering your own personal connection to source, in whatever form it may take, it is imperative to first release and let go of any tired or distorted paradigms. These old tapes may not even be yours and chances are, they may no longer serve you.

"A perfect example of this is my beautiful daughter. Ever since she was born and even in my belly, she has witnessed my practice of yoga and meditation. She has also had some strong Jewish influences in her life. Yet today she has no interest in any of it. I am often asked if she practices yoga. The answer is a resounding no. She hikes and swims. As a parent, I observe this and realize she is forming her own identity. I certainly do not feel it is my job to force her into any spiritual discipline. My gift is allowing her the freedom to choose her own path." ~ Miranda

As you step fully into your life power, including this potent and auspicious realm of spirit, it is imperative for the wise gown up version of yourself to be present to make the choices. For this to be possible, the wounds and distortions from the past need to be gently and lovingly forgiven and transformed into the true authentic expression of who you are today. One of the most vital qualities of being a woman fully embodying her power is the ability to receive. Without a doorway into the realm of the spiritual, you may be living life without receiving all the bounty, synchronicities and seeming miracles that this unseen world has to offer.

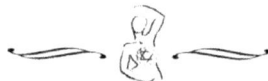

"A human being is a citizen of two worlds,
inner and outer, and one must develop the ability
to access both worlds without any confusion."
~ Swami Rama

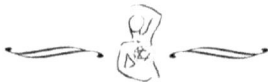

TWO WORLDS COLLIDE

Random thoughts of madness dancing with devotion.

I long for you like a child for its mother.
A yearning deep in my bones to belong to you again.
My sins fully absolved dissolving back into unity by the void of the whole.
My separateness no longer a razors edge. Splintering the fringes of existence.
No longer abiding by the rules. No more deciding on who I have to be today.
No more longing. No more rips and tears. Just a simple reconciliation with the one.

"But what about me?" cried the ego
"If we go home and unite with source I will die.
Where will all my colors go if I reunite with only light?
I will lose all my spectrum, my prism, myself. I will no longer be unique or special
I will not even exist. I want to be me. I demand my own identity.

Come eat with me. Drink with me.
Dance with me in memories past and future dreams and fears.
In my world of separateness. In my realm of independence.

No, not in the light
In the shadows where I can still dim
The insurmountable awareness and remain unconscious.
"I do not want to go home yet. Let us stay a while," the ego cooed to the soul.

And the soul gently responded,
"Let go little one. Surrender.
All will be revealed and remembered.
There is nothing to fear.
Nothing will die.

Only the story of you.
Then you will become me.
Infinite boundless energy and light
An emergence of the infinite potential which resides within us all.

Come fly with me.
Come dance in the flame of eternal existence.
I pray for reconciliation."

And yet, the two worlds continued to collide...

TO THINE OWN SELF BE TRUE

"I am the captain of my fate,
the master of my soul."
~ William Ernest Henley

As you meander or bulldoze through this journey called life, it is vital to remember that you are the writer, director, main actor and stage manager. You get to decide the flavor, actions and adventures of your experience. This may leave you with a deep resounding sense of responsibility. Yet to realize that you can transform and manifest your life in any way you choose, can also redeem you with a feeling of power, fortitude and freedom.

From this perspective, you can then observe your life and inquire:

◈ Are you playing out your existence in a way that is authentic and aligned with your truth?

◈ Or are you in a job or situation that has nothing to do with your divine purpose or relationships that are forcing you to lie?

The good news is spirituality can play a major role in aiding you to live an authentic and honest life filled with moments of joy, silence, reverence, gratitude and beauty.

Spirituality by its very nature invokes a passageway back to the self.

When you respect your truth, you may well decide that your health and well-being is of the utmost importance. This might lead to you canceling a commitment or two, therefore allowing you to relax and replenish if needed. Rest can be extremely healing in and of itself. Or it might be that you choose to add in a quality that has been seriously ignored for a while, such as sensuality, no timeline or outrageous fun. Any choice you make to align with taking care of the physical body and elevating it out of survival mode will open many of the doorways to spirituality.

"Being self employed, I am sometimes in awe about what I have orchestrated for myself in a single day. My image that I am a 'wonder woman with a to-do list' certainly dictates some of the decisions and art directing in this play of mine. What is fascinating is that I have no one else at whom to point the finger. I chose it, I organized it and I said yes to it. I must say that as I live the teachings of 'A Woman's Truth' I do have less and less days or weeks of insane unconscious behavior." ~ Miranda

You are the captain of your vessel. At any moment you get to choose which way to turn, respond, act or react. What is also clear is that other people's lives are not under your stage management or script, even though it is sometimes tempting to become the dictator of someone else's life, instead of the director of your own play.

Yet you are in control of how you choose to react to another person's choices or dilemmas. Your seat is the one where your truth is honored. You can choose not to participate if you do not like the circumstances. Your place in the audience can be changed if you are not enjoying the view. You may not be able to remove the very tall, noisy, popcorn-eating person in front of you, but you can choose to move to another chair on the other side of the theater.

"I am always amazed at how I sometimes struggle to change the physical arena I find myself in. It could be the location of a restaurant table that is not working or someone's body being in too close a proximity to mine. In the past, I have literally felt myself squirm in reaction before acting on changing the situation. Yet today, with a commitment to living in my own truth, I will ask for a different table or literally remove myself from a situation. Ah... freedom at last!" ~ Miranda

SPIRITUALITY VERSUS RELIGION

In a world with such diverse religions,
are they not all singing the same song?

Spirituality is a very large and encompassing subject and it can certainly get lost in translation. Traditionally religions have regarded spirituality as an integral aspect of a religious experience. Yet nowadays there is a much broader view. Interestingly, there was certainly a plethora of spiritual practices before many religions came into being. What is being brought to light here is that spirituality has a life of its own that does not need to be connected to or aligned with any religion. From this viewpoint, spiritual practices are not to be mistaken for religious or cultural teachings. Yet they can walk hand in hand quite beautifully.

Many words are used to speak of the realm of spirituality: Divine, mystical, sacred, source of inspiration, stillness, introspection, incorporeal, contemplation are just a few. The following is an offering of one possible definition and how spiritual qualities can be translated into your daily existence:

Through introspection, contemplation and practices an inner life is developed and nurtured, which animates the body and mind, allowing a Higher Spiritual perspective to be revealed. By choosing to live by the elevated realms of love, hope and awareness, one's behavior aligns with being of service to your own potential and purpose and the Highest good of all other beings involved.

An everyday translation of this would be a heavenly win-win.

For some, a quiet moment to meditate and center yourself is a spiritual practice. For others, spending time in nature or participating in an activity you love will ignite the inner world. There are many ways to nourish your soul. Whatever you do to quiet your mind and relax your being is considered a connection to the world of mysticism.

INTERACTIONS OF LOVE, TIME, MONEY OR ENERGY:

◆ In these situations, it is about releasing all judgment regarding what this win-win should look like.

◆ Then handing it over to the creative and boundless supply of energy that resides in the universe.

◆ The human responsibility is to be present and conscious enough to know if the situation at hand is ultimately right action.

◆ Once this is discerned, the spiritual realm can then take care of exactly how this plays out, what helpful and beneficial people need to be involved and what synchronicities need to happen.

◆ Ending with the result of the miraculous outcome prayed for.

In other words, as you give your very best in all good consciousness, you can surrender the rest of the outcome to the realms of Spirit.

"I would say that I am a deeply spiritual person. My work is spiritual and my home is one big living altar (my poor housekeeper!) I practice meditation and energy work daily. I pray and I choose to honor this aspect of myself as much as my physical mundane form. Yet when someone said to me how she wished she had my kind of faith, I was struck by my response. I explained that I have grappled with the concept of faith my whole life: I wished I could drop into the blind world of belief where I see others.

After many years, I am still no closer to being engulfed in a religious faith than when I was confirmed at age nine having no real feeling about the experience. Yet I do have a knowing that I am part of a whole. I am a tiny drop in this huge expansive energy of the universe. That in this moment and incarnation, I manifested in all my glory and pitfalls! I believe there has to be an intelligence behind the creation of this earth and universe because it is so miraculous, beautiful and all encompassing.

The more I study the human body in relationship to nutrition and health, the more I am in awe of its magnificence and ability to heal. It seems as though everything is programmed for survival. As I watch a sunset or a full moon rise, again I am awestruck by the exquisite details and miracles of this place we call home.

Is this faith?

From my perception I acknowledge that some energy force, much bigger and greater than me, is behind all of creation and in the same breath, all of destruction. My choice in this lifetime is to find as many ways as possible to connect to this infinite boundless sea of energy. In this space, I remember I am never alone. I cannot be because my drop of energy called Miranda is a part of this nectar, this ocean, this miracle of the universe." ~ Miranda

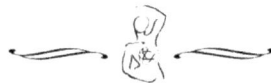

"To find the way, close your eyes, listen closely, and attend with your heart."

~ Anonymous

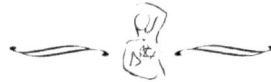

THE WEAKEST LINK

We are only as strong as our weakest link.

Unfortunately, living in the western world, spirituality is often the weakest link. In many eastern countries, spiritual practice dominates life. Yet in the west a devotional existence is certainly not encouraged, let alone a way of being. Taking basic care of the material form is often easier because of its ability to physically respond with pain or symptom, yet even this can be forgotten. Paying attention to the mind is programmed at a very early age as a way to get what you need. You may have noticed, your emotions can sometimes overflow like a tidal wave whether you like it or not. These three aspects of the Self tend to be realized, acknowledged and taken care of, even if on a very basic, fundamental level.

In comparison, spirituality can easily be ignored. Days can go by being practical, taking care of the mundane and the details, yet never allowing a glimpse of the unseen world to unveil itself. You could say that this world of spirit actually needs to be invited in, given space and consciously invoked into your daily life. In contrast, spirituality is often only used in desperation.

When a disaster happens, then you fall to your knees and pray. Yet, while life is ticking along, the mention of God or a higher power can be neglected for days.

With an awareness of this dynamic, it would seem appropriate to encourage this weak link to be strengthened. The world of the unseen needs to be nurtured to stay alive. This can be done by consciously choosing to invite the sacred into your life on a daily basis, however this translates to you.

HERE ARE SOME SIMPLE SPIRITUAL WAYS OF BEING:

As you consciously choose to embody some of these qualities, your spiritual connection will become galvanized, helping to unveil your true purpose and mission here on earth.

◆ **What is your spiritual way of being?**

◊ A prayer

◊ A deep sense of gratitude for your life

◊ A meditation or Yoga Nidra

◊ Time in nature or planting your feet in the earth

◊ Being of service or connecting to your spiritual community

◊ Silence or stillness

◊ Taking a few deep breaths

◊ Giving and receiving love

◊ Dancing or listening to music

◊ Laughter, joy, awe, wonder

◊ Surrender or acceptance

◊ Feel free to add your personal spiritual truth

A SPIRITUAL MOMENT

By pausing and becoming present and conscious
of the moment, the mundane can transform
into the miraculous.

How often have you gone through your day trudging through the lists and demands with your head down, your will strong and a heavy weight in your heart?

In fact, empty days can reoccur unless you consciously pause long enough to invite in the essence of joy, creativity or love. One imbalance in life occurs when you become overwhelmingly busy. In these times, the tendency is to pull on your masculine presence to take over and demand it to take control of the stress, which can cause rather a bulldozer effect. In this situation, there is no pause or space for your feminine to enhance your life or to invoke spirituality, beauty or delight.

The beauty is that literally any moment or wrinkle in time can become spiritual or filled with amazement, by simply changing your point of view from the mundane to the miraculous. Just as a photographer will change a lens, you too can invoke a new perspective by pausing for a moment and becoming quiet. You are then open to perceive the world and miracles around you. As you may have realized, you do need to look up into the vast sky to notice a rainbow or the beauty of the moon.

Allow your viewfinder to expand and to open to the intricate beauties all around you. However hard your day, there is always wonder and miracles present. Even in those moments where you feel pinned in a difficult situation and literally feel as though there is no way out. Remember, your heart is still beating, the breath still functioning and you are always loved. The sun is still setting, the moon is still rising and nature is still adorned in all her ruthlessness and glory and behind the clouds, the sun is shining.

Sometimes you may find yourself stuck with some pretty harsh or demanding tapes playing in your head. At this moment, it is vital to expand your horizon to one of a spiritual nature to invoke the love and guidance of this unseen infinite world.

It really is as simple as asking for help.

"I have often wondered why prayer seems to work. From the rather logical side of my brain I realize that when I do pray, I am pausing the momentum of my life, which is causing me stress and changing my outlook to call on a realm that has infinite possibilities and solutions. In that moment, I am surrendering myself as a mere little mortal having to fix what seems to be an unfathomable situation. In this exchange my mind relaxes, my body quiets, my breath resumes and it is as though I get to start the race again, yet this time with a sense of support and help from the universe." ~ Miranda

RAISING YOUR SPIRITS

How to incorporate spirituality into your daily life.

For some, spirituality is a calling from dawn till dusk. Meaning they live in a monastery or have a strong affiliation to a church or spiritual teachings. In this situation, time does not have to be made for their spiritual practices because they are lived day by day. Yet unless you have chosen to be a nun or a spiritual guide in this lifetime, the chances are your lifestyle will not necessarily support an encounter with the world of the sacred on a daily basis.

Yet for the rest of humanity whose lives of 'chop wood and carry water' have become so busy and mundane, the idea of spending time doing one more task can just about tip you over the edge.

The question is how to incorporate spirituality into an already hectic way of life. Before the *how* is delved into, it seems as though the *why* needs to be clarified first.

◆ What are the benefits of carving out a portion of your day that will not get your work done, the dishes washed, the kids or cleaning picked up and certainly does not cook dinner?

A good question indeed.

"In my own personal experience, if I meditate and walk each morning, I encounter a very different kind of day than if I do not. During this time, I set my intentions that are all about me. I take this time to fill, center and prepare myself for the day ahead. Life still happens, but how I perceive and react is certainly calmer and less explosive if I have done some sort of spiritual practice that morning. It is as though the essence of this inward motion fills my well and reserve tank. The bottom line is I know how vital it is to replenish my spirit and refill this well daily. Or else I will literally be running on fumes and we all know how ugly and stressful that can be. By committing to this precious window each morning, I find I do not take life quite so seriously. The part of me who can observe and witness this exquisite yet sometimes brutal play of life is strengthened and I have a constant reminder throughout the day that this experience is just one aspect of who I am." ~ Miranda

Connecting up to the spiritual aspect of yourself will change the lens you see through. By seeping yourself in spiritual practices which resonate with the core of your being, life is then filtered with this spiritual essence, turning fear into faith, frustration into patience, judgment into compassion and envy into abundance.

Our greatest source of power is not in our muscles, but in our thoughts. By changing your mind, you can change your life.

Connecting to the creative source of existence will encourage more spiritual moments throughout the day. You may have noticed that when you were pregnant, you saw bellies everywhere or when you were thinking about buying a new car, you suddenly saw that particular make on every street corner. It is the same with spirituality. As you become more spiritual, this world of the sacred will be attracted to you like a magnet. Even without thinking, you will notice a beautiful cloud formation, pausing to enjoy this moment in all its glory and beauty.

In every instance there is potential to live in the spiritual essence of love or the human aspect of fear. To choose the doorway of love takes courage which comes from the heart. Every time you are engulfed in fear, your survival is being threatened on some level. As you reach this poignant crossroad, you can choose either to succumb to the reptilian aspect of the brain or to elevate yourself to the divine connection of source. This seems like another valid reason to invite some devotion, stillness and prayer into your life.

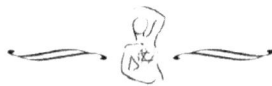

"Courage is fear that has learned how to pray."
~ Anonymous

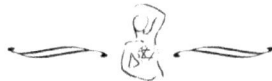

Now that you know why spirituality will enhance and support you, the following suggestions will help to guide you in forming a practice of your own.

HOW TO BRING SPIRITUALITY INTO YOUR LIFE:

◆ **The early morning, even before getting up and dressed, is an auspicious time to connect to your own personal spirituality and practices.**
There is great value in carving out time for your spiritual practice early in the day; otherwise, life tends to eclipse this precious opportunity.

◆ **A few moments of stillness and silence are literally golden.**

◆ **A prayer can be done at any moment and in any situation.**

◆ **Gratitude always fills your being bringing you back to center.**
Being thankful invokes a feeling of being at least half-full to overflowing, if not more, setting the tone and flavor for the day ahead.

◆ **Take a moment to remember who you really are.**
An extraordinary, timeless being residing in this miracle called a body.

THE SPIRIT OF LOVE

*Just because you love or forgive someone
does not mean you have to have them in your life.*

In the precious movement of loving yourself, you receive the bounty of your own love. This simple act will fill, nourish and replenish your whole being. From this overflow, the gift is that you have plenty of love and energy to go around and freely give to others without any resistance or resentment.

Unfortunately, this is not as simple as it sounds when you have been deeply hurt, rejected or betrayed by someone you love.

This scenario then poses the question: How do you balance respecting, honoring and taking care of yourself and still keep an open heart for the love you feel for someone who has hurt you?

One solution is to realize that you can still love this person, yet you do have a choice as to what kind of relationship to be in with them.

"In my own personal experience, I have noticed how I shut my heart down as a way to protect myself. Even though a torrent of emotions may be flooding my body, I have a strange ability to remain calm and cool. I am a little like the 'Ice Queen', when faced with the culprit, whom I deemed has caused me harm. It feels as though to keep the flow of love going in that moment will hurt me even more. It seems too vulnerable, too painful and a part of me screams, 'They no longer deserve my love!'

As I shut down my heart, an interesting occurrence happens. I also seem to shut down my capacity to connect to the person and receive their love. As I stifle my ability to feel and hold the twist in place, I have come to realize how I am ultimately damaging myself with this action. As I cease the flow of love and compassion to another, I am also shutting down the gift of love to myself. There have been people in my life who have caused me harm, yet I still feel a heartfelt connection, even though I may not like, respect or want them around.

At this juncture, I am happy to say I have enough self-respect and love to choose not to have contact with them yet still keep my heart open. There will always be an aspect of myself who wants to be spiteful and get revenge. In the past, I would deliver this punishment by blocking the flow of my love. However, I now realize there is another way. I can keep my heart open, yet still take care of my own being by being clear about how I choose to interact with the person. By loving myself, I am no longer placed in jeopardy." ~ Miranda

There are many choices in speaking your truth as a courageous act of self-love:

◆ Define a new relationship.

◆ Let them know if they cannot treat you with love and respect, you can no longer associate with them.

◆ Limit contact with them.

◆ Only have contact a certain way (such as email).

◆ Not talk to them face to face.

◆ Not see them anymore.

◆ Have no contact with them at all.

When someone is lying or disrespecting you, choose one of the following:

◆ "When you can talk to me with respect, we can have a conversation."

◆ "When you can treat me with love and respect, we can have a relationship."

◆ "When you can be respectful and honest with me, we can spend time together."

From this vantage point, you are being clear, respectful and will remain in your power. You are having a conversation from the heart, not the mind or the ego. It is then up to the other person to see if they are willing or able to step up to a new level of relationship. This ultimately sets you free and allows you to surround yourself with people who truly do love, respect and support you.

When you keep the flame of love alive in your heart, you will remain balanced and authentic. It does not mean you allow yourself to be walked on or disrespected. You will clarify this by stating the new terms of the relationship.

Choose to come from a place of love, rather than one of anger, hurt or rage. These latter emotions tend to ignite a reaction of fear, rather than a conscious act of love.

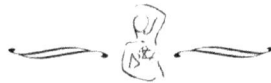

"Your task is not to seek for love,
but merely to seek and find all the barriers
within yourself that you have built against it."
~ Rumi

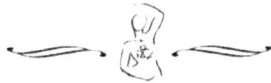

THE ULTIMATE FREEDOM

For~give~ness.

*H*ave you ever noticed that the word *give* is at the center of for*give*ness? Therefore, when you choose to forgive you are ultimately giving a precious gift to yourself and to the other person involved. As you give up the grievance, which dishonored you, your psyche will naturally rise to a higher level of consciousness and come from a place of love, rather than survival.

Forgiving yourself is the ultimate act of self-love. The greatest choice you can make is to forgive all your past decisions, behaviors and regrets. Imagine being as loving, kind and compassionate to yourself as you would a young child or a dear friend that you deeply care for. This is a lesson in generosity and remembering you are always worthy of love and deserve forgiveness as much as anyone else.

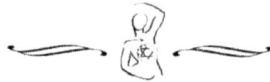

"We are all children of the universe, of creation, of Source.
Thus said, the most potent elixir and cure you can give to any malady
will always be your own well and capacity to love and forgive yourself."
~ Anonymous

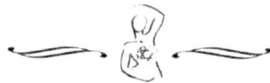

The foundation of 'Living a Spiritual Life' is the practice of self-love and forgiveness. Once this core is established, it is then time to forge ahead to forgive those you are still holding hostage or ransom. In these scenarios, you are spending your time and energy keeping these people and situations alive and captured within you. You are the guard, the judge, the gatekeeper, the jury and the wounded victim all rolled into one. This is a heavy load and price to pay. Especially when love and forgiveness are literally free and have no baggage or weight associated with them.

"One day a strange belief arose from my subconscious. I was moving the body and allowing a deep sense of stillness to overflow my mind. In the release from the usual chatter, a guttural voice from my childhood tore through my being, bleeding with grief over the statement that if someone really loved me, they would never hurt or cause me harm. This limited belief has haunted me my whole life because in reality, many of the people who dearly love me have caused me heartache and pain.

By recognizing and honoring this belief, I am now still free to let people love me. Yet I also know from a wiser perspective, they can always hurt me. The good news is that I now have the tools and knowledge to always love, honor and respect myself, therefore not causing myself harm. This is the ultimate love affair!" ~ Miranda

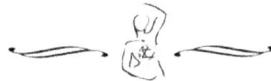

"It is easy to take liberty for granted, when you have never had it taken from you."
~ Anonymous

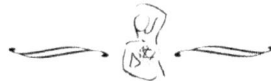

A LETTER OF TRUTH

The intention of these letters is freedom, not revenge.

Have you ever been in a situation with a person where the pathways of communication have sunk to such an all time low, that it seems impossible for a solution to be reached? This scenario can be extremely painful and if left unresolved, could cause harm by the stress stored in some part of your being, festering away.

When you write a letter of truth, the intention is for you to put pen to paper, rant and rave until there is nothing left to throw up. The brilliance is any venom, poison or curses you may be spewing at the other person are lost in translation because no one actually gets to read the letter, apart from you. It is your own personal testimony, feelings and truth in that moment. The healing occurs as you give yourself an opening to purge, releasing the torrent of emotions that have been building within you.

The letter is then burnt as an offering to release any of the anger, pain or rage. This in turn sets you free from the past, the situation and the people involved.

This simple process of writing an honest, soulful or outraged letter to someone is a powerful and effective way to store the pain or feelings in your own being no longer.

"I myself have had many miraculous results using 'Letters of Truth'. The biggest redemption is when the person or situation no longer bothers me. Sometimes though, it may take more than one letter! I have also received unprompted apologies unexpectedly. As you release the rope of hatred, the other person has nothing to pull on. This means the situation has to change and in my experience, a tug of war is tiring, hard work and can leave you face down in the mud!" ~ Miranda

WRITING A LETTER OF TRUTH:

◈ Carve out some quiet time so you will not be disturbed or distracted.

◈ Sit with a pen and paper and conjure up an image of the person.
   This will help you connect to the truth and feelings surrounding the situation.

◈ Simply begin to write.

◈ Do not censer yourself.
   Emotions may come up. This is good. Swearing is encouraged! Your handwriting may become illegible, which is fine as no one is going to read it.

◈ Write and write until there is nothing left to say.

◈ When complete, burn the letter. As the paper burns, ask that there is a complete healing between you and the person or situation.

◈ Ask for the outcome to be for everyone's highest good and let go of any agenda or specific outcome.
   This will allow the ego to release being right and will invite miracles.

◈ See your emotions, pains, hurts, abandonments, rejections, denials, jealousies and defenses all dissolve in the fire and literally go up in smoke.
   They say that smoke is a sign of releasing karma, which is all-good! Give thanks and gratitude for the blessings you will receive from holding onto the past and your vendetta no longer. This will literally make space in you for new beginnings and more love.

◈ You may feel like writing more than one letter.
   There is no limit and you will know when you are done because you will literally have nothing left to say.

"It would not be in your best interest to set up a scenario where you could accidentally or unconsciously send the letter. Therefore, I would encourage you not to type it as an email. I have known this to happen and although the ultimate outcome was good, the tornado that ensued could have possibly caused more harm than good." ~ Miranda

FILLING IN YOUR CIRCLE

The road less traveled.

When you choose to live in your own center and circle of intimate space, you will gain a new perspective. From this vantage point, it will become crystal clear if the energy you are surrounding yourself with is for your highest good. Without having a strong attachment to your authentic essence, you may well find yourself dancing around the periphery of your life. From this cliff's edge, it is easy to be drawn into the turbulence of the world below, allowing your job, relationships and any other daily occurrences to pull you off your mark. This can place you in a constant state of stress or need of repair.

As you spend time realizing your intention to stay aligned with your midpoint, it is vital to discern what will help you stay centered and connected to your own pool of serenity. Once this is established, it will then create a strong foundation for your true essence to ripple out into the periphery of your life.

AUTHENTICALLY ALIGNING WITH YOUR CENTER:

◈ As you may recall, one of the qualities that widens and stabilizes your center is the strength and clarity of your own **truth**. The more you recognize, honor and practice living from your authenticity, the wider and stronger the central platform becomes. Your own sphere of light and integrity expands with each truth, action and decision made from this place of honesty. When practiced daily this truth telling will invoke a vibrant confidence, which will deeply affect your ability to be in intimate relationships. As you live from your genuine self, you will be clear whether it is appropriate to invite someone into your inner sanctuary or to allow them to touch the edges of your circle.

◈ By living in strong relationship with 'The Foundational Trinity' you will get enough rest, good food and exercise which serves in keeping you balanced and living from your center.

◈ Choosing to say **no** when appropriate will ward off spending energy you do not have, will keep your boundaries clear and your sense of self aligned.

◆ Nurturing and listening to your **Feminine, Masculine, Child** and **Self** will help keep them all in good order, which will also benefit you by maintaining your center.

◆ It seems appropriate that '**Loving Yourself**' would fill in many of the cracks.

◆ The circle of your life can also be deeply filled with **Spirituality** by facilitating a relationship with spiritual practices and the unseen world.

Ponder what your world of spirituality looks or feels like.

It could be as simple as a prayer sent, an intention set, a meditation, a moment of stillness or being in recognition of a Higher Power. These are all potent pathways to fill your circle. Another beautiful way to invite spirituality into this energy field is to play with the messages and symbols that life is always doling out. Sometimes answers to a request, question or inspiration may come in the most unusual ways.

"One of my most intuitive places where I receive high frequency information from my Higher Self is often in the shower!" ~ Miranda

By being open to the signs, messages, gentle and not so gentle nudges from the energetic realm, a completely new arena of guidance becomes apparent. It is by pausing the fast pace of life that the missed turn is revealed. As it is said:

"Be still and know God."

"It was an interesting weekend. As I was preparing to go away, a toilet started to leak and a shower backed up. Then on the way, my car needed coolant. All the issues seemed to be about water leaking all over the place. At this point in my life I do tend to pay attention to signs, so I did spend a moment reigning myself in and settling back into my own sense of existence. However, it seemed as though the play was not over. I finally arrived at my destination. The next morning, a large decorative fairy had fallen nose first into the dirt outside and had broken her wing. Then a bird flew into the house. Not an hour later, a pigeon fell from the sky like a thunderbolt at my feet. Very dazed and confused it walked over to a corner. At this point, I took a sigh of relief because these kinds of events do seem to happen in threes and the message, well it seemed pretty loud and clear. Life is scary and hurts if you do not have wings to fly high enough to see the birds-eye view. I was spending the weekend figuring out how to pay for my daughter's college, which may well have clipped my wings out of financial fear. Basically at the point of the pigeon falling from heaven, I started to pray!" ~ Miranda

Staying awake to spiritual gifts and messages can be highly amusing and obscure, yet extremely enlightening. By remaining grateful and listening to the blessings in disguise, you may even be nudged in a better direction, deflecting a possible head-on collision of your own.

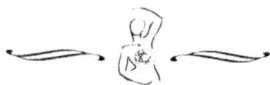

"The winds of grace blow all the time.
All we need to do is set sail."

~ Anonymous

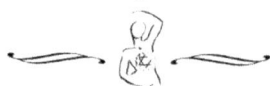

As you incorporate spirituality into your life, it can bring about a sense of peace and calm. Thus allowing you to decide clearly what the right course of action might be, rather than being dictated to by the realms of other people's desires and needs. Again, this is about staying in your center and power and responding from this place of poise.

Imagine yourself curled up in front of a cozy fire, in a big armchair with a soft blanket and a cup of hot tea. From this vantage point, if a huge storm began to break, chances are you would not run out in the freezing cold rain unless you had to. Yet you may enjoy the lightening through the window. Because your center is calm on the inside, the outside chaos and drama seemed unappealing and it is easy to stay where you are. However, if your inner world is in turmoil with chaos, fighting, leaking roofs and drama, then the outside storm may seem like a sanctuary. At least the rain does not answer back, although the thunder may.

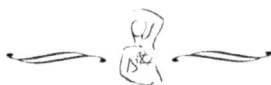

"There is more to life than.
increasing its speed."
~ Gandhi

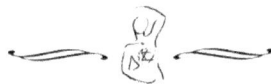

MUNDANE OR MIRACULOUS?

You Choose.

A spiritual practice can be invoked simple by the state of your consciousness. In life, there is always a choice. A task can be viewed and lived out as a chore. This usually means it is to be accomplished as quickly as possible; with no reverence and a mechanical get it done approach is instigated. This translates into the world of the mundane. In comparison, the exact same task can be completed with a sense of awe and wonder. If while accomplishing the chore, you choose to be present and conscious of the touch, feel, sight or sounds surrounding the experience, everything changes. How often have you looked up to witness a butterfly or a beautiful sky and paused in that moment to bask in its beauty? As soon as you become present and open to miracles, the same ordinary task can be transformed from a 'to do list' experience to one that can add joy and quality to this journey called life.

A perfect example of this is the activity of going for a walk.

The practical reason for going on a walk is probably to exercise, stay healthy or lose weight. These are all perfectly valid. With this intention and probably a tight timeline, you march out of the house with your watch and power walk (maybe!) your way around the neighborhood. It is as though you have stepped into a tunnel and the world around you is devoid of any beauty. It is very annoying to have to wait for a passing car and why do people want to stop and chat? The conversation in your head is traveling as fast as your feet and it seems as though many voices are talking at once, problem solving, worrying and trying to figure out the day ahead.

You get a good view of the road as you watch your footing and get back just in time to shower and be ready for the day. Next task...mission accomplished.

Scenario two has the same purpose but with an added aspect; to actually enjoy the experience and stop to smell the roses, as they say. Instead of this being a purely physical activity, you choose to take care of your mental, emotional and spiritual bodies.

"My morning walk is actually a 'two for one'. My body moves, but along the way I pray, set my intentions, practice Reiki on myself and loved ones or talk if I am with one of my dear friends. They say what you talk or think about as you stride along becomes reality as the crisscrossing motion of the arms and legs helps to manifest your words and thoughts. Therefore, I am conscious not to let my mind or talk ramble too far into the swamps of my wounds or insecurities. By the end of my walk I feel centered and balanced on a physical, mental, emotional and spiritual level and my day moves forward with this flavor. Thank God!" ~ Miranda

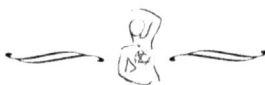

"Ask, and it will be given you;
seek, and you will find; knock, and it will be opened to you."

~ Jesus

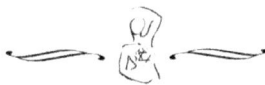

TIME AND SPIRITUALITY

why be in such a hurry to meet a deadline?

The beauty of being connected to the world of spirituality and energy is that in these realms, time does not exist or matter. As you have noticed, the imagination can effortlessly travel forward or back, immaterial of the timeline. This same gift arises as you perform spiritual practices, allowing the part of the mind that controls time to let go and relax. In this space, a minute can seem like an hour or vice versa. When you are connected to the essence of yourself as a spiritual being, there is a remembering that a part of you is immortal and therefore time has no real reference or meaning.

Obviously, as a human being, it is sometimes appropriate or even vital to follow a schedule. There are situations when willpower, the linear masculine brain or tension will be the cultivating factor demanding a very specific course of action in a limited space of time. This is fine for short periods of stress. Yet, on a regular basis, following the rhythms of nature is a much sweeter way.

"Each year around the fall I tend to get sick. It would seem as though I am not practicing what I preach enough! To slow down, go inward, hibernate and enjoy the more relaxed pace as the fall changes into winter. Strangely, I get extremely annoyed at still having to achieve as much during this season, as I do naturally want to change my pace and do less. My body then dictates the desire to connect with the rhythm of nature because my mind will not succumb. Hopefully I am learning this lesson!" ~ Miranda

YIELD TO THE RHYTHM AND WISDOM OF NATURE:

◆ Allow yourself to relax and slow down once the sun sets.

◆ Wake up as the sun rises.

◆ Break the fast of a night's sleep by eating a healthy, nutritious breakfast.

◆ Cleanse and energize yourself during the spring and summer and slow down and rejuvenate during the fall and winter.

◆ Try experiencing a day without a clock, computer or any other time line.
This can be as delicious and juicy as a pajama day and invokes the feminine.

Just as the rhythms of nature dictates, a seed is best planted in the spring, where it receives light, water and nourishment throughout the summer. Fall is the time to harvest all you have planted before. As fall turns to winter, it is not the time of year to sow new seeds as the ground lies still and fallow. The seasons of fall and winter are a part of the decay and destruction cycles of life. In the stillness and lack of growth, space is made for new seeds, intentions and dreams to arise from the dormancy and be fostered in the spring that follows. This cycle is stronger, more powerful and potent than any thought in your mind to try to be a spring flower in the depths and darkness of winter. Nature in all of her wisdom and infinite cycles will always win. Rather than fighting with the source of your creation, bow to her rhythm, become a part of her cycle and allow her to support your dreams.

"It was a stressful week and somehow I had manifested three huge deadlines in my life. At one point in desperation, I said aloud "I hate deadlines." I then stopped because I really heard the word, 'deadline.' Suddenly it felt ominous and lethal. Was I slowly welcoming death by having all these set times that I believed would be the demise of me if I did not follow? I have now chosen not to use this phrase anymore and attempt not to give myself such unreachable goals. Yet there are still days when I look at my calendar and realize I have no one else to blame. If I did have a boss that had given me this list, I would seriously think she was an unreasonable bitch! Although my mind struggles with surrender, I do know it will feed my body, my being and my soul." ~ Miranda

The aspect of the mind that controls time is linear, masculine and very connected to survival and the mundane everyday world. It cannot comprehend infinity nor the concept of what is behind the universe. It gets boggled or overwhelmed by such thoughts and resorts back to the mundane. When you meditate, pray, become still or deeply relaxed, this aspect of the mind gets a vacation and the ability to rise into the spiritual realms is amplified and enhanced.

"As a child I would ask my Dad daily what was behind the stars, the sun and the black sky. Mind you, I was asking a highly intelligent civil engineer and atheist. He would explain galaxies and constellations and then I would ask, what was beyond them. In his frustration, he would have to answer infinity. What was infinity, I then wanted to know, and on and on. He could not give me a logical answer and would finally have to respond that he did not know." ~ Miranda

SPIRITUALITY AND STILLNESS

It is in the pause that we are able to receive.

*I*magine a drop of continuous nectar gently falling into the crown of your head. This essence is a gift of energy, guidance, nourishment and light being given to you in every moment of every day. It is as though the ambrosia of the universe is perpetually supporting you. To receive this blessing all you need to do is be is still enough to allow it to fall into your essence. Yet if you are running too fast the drop will still flow, but you will have missed the gift by being too far ahead. Both stillness and silence allow you to receive blessings and support on many levels and even the odd miracle.

A Journey Into Present Moment:

◆ Choose an activity that you do on a regular basis.
It could range from flossing your teeth, to taking a bath, to paying your bills.

◆ Accomplish this activity without a timeline.
As you know, the clock does not run spirituality.

◆ Now, instead of bulldozing your way through this task or becoming completely unconscious, take all the time in the world.
How often have you arrived at your destination and had very little memory of the actual drive there? This is unconsciousness at its best, or worst!

◆ Set your intention to find a sense of joy and pleasure in what you are doing.
This will mean being conscious and present in the moment.

◆ Let go of there being a result.
This will allow you to enjoy the experience as part of the journey of life, rather than judging whether you removed an item off the 'to-do' list.

◆ Breathe.
Allow your body to relax and notice the miraculous details of life around you.

◆ Enjoy the moments of this exercise.

◆ Notice how you feel at the end.

By bringing spirituality into your daily life, you will allow the pause and space to receive energy and any blessings that might be just hovering, waiting to be given. Think of the white rabbit in 'Alice in Wonderland'. He is the perfect depiction of no time to be still. When you are on the run like this, there is actually no space to receive either.

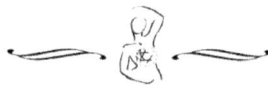

"Through return to simple living comes control of desire.
In control of desires, stillness is attained.
In stillness the world is restored."

~ Lao Tzu

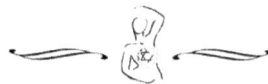

HOW TO KNOW GOD

what is your own personal temple or church?

Often the world of spirituality is depicted by images of being on your knees or your legs crossed, having to be quiet, still, calm or with your eyes closed. Well, try telling that to a gospel singer! All that energy, sound and vitality is certainly very different from quiet, yet it is filled to overflowing with a connection to a higher power.

Many people are drawn to connect
to their spiritual side through the physical body.

Spirituality is an intensely personal experience and difficult to put into words. There is no right or wrong here. For one person the prospect of running up a mountain would be their idea of hell. For another, it gets them closer to the higher realms. The point is to find the movement, sound or activity that has the ability to transform you from your mundane existence into a space of being utterly lost in the present moment. The freedom this allows is that you no longer care what anybody else thinks, what you look like or how you are acting. In these moments, the Higher Self eclipses the ego in a glorious, wondrous and liberating experience.

POSSIBLE AVENUES TO SPIRITUALITY:

◆ Dancing	◆ Wailing	◆ Sex	◆ Writing
◆ Drumming	◆ Crying	◆ Bikes	◆ Gardening
◆ Running	◆ Chanting	◆ Food	◆ Swimming
◆ Hiking	◆ Laughing	◆ Art	◆ Animals
◆ Surfing	◆ Music	◆ Films	◆ Hugging
◆ Cycling	◆ Poetry	◆ Cooking	◆ Conversations
◆ Skiing	◆ Instruments	◆ Playing	◆ Rock Climbing
◆ Singing	◆ Gongs	◆ Reading	◆ Nature

Seriously, the list is endless.

The question to ask here is:

◆ What is your way to connect to the Spiritual aspect of life?

And even more importantly:

◆ Are you living this way in your life?

WHAT YOU SEEK IS SEEKING YOU

"Every journey begins with a single step."

*E*very time you set an intention, have a dream, make a wish or a say a prayer, you take a step towards this vision and in response, these goals take a step towards you.

Eventually the two shall meet.

The key here is patience. Often it can take time for an idea or a creation to manifest into material form. Rather than focusing so hard on the out and out destination or result, it is vital to remember how every single step, phone call, smile or action may well be another stride on the path. This then allows the journey of the manifestation to become an important part of the experience. For an inspiration to be birthed, the energy of creation needs to be present and the event can often be a labor filled experience. As you may have noticed, even when the project or invention is born, it will still need to be parented for many years to come.

"I remember my first book being published. Five years in the making and it seemed as though the last piece was the hardest part. Yet my book was complete. Hundreds of copies of my creation surrounded me. I had ISBN numbers and all. After relishing in this achievement, it did not take me long to realize the journey had really only just begun. I now had to market and had to sell my book. To this day, I am still involved in nurturing, promoting and signing this beloved creation!" ~ Miranda

Everyone has brilliant and extraordinary brain waves and ideas. Yet if these inspirational concepts stay lodged in the virtual brain, the creation will never be held in your hands. To bring a vision into form it begins with one step. It could be sharing the idea with someone or calling the person who has the right contact for you.

"I personally seem to have the opposite problem. My virtual brain never stops with new ideas, concepts and visions for my home, my business or myself. With each new idea, I am like an excited child trying to catch a butterfly. I will then make the call or buy the materials, whatever it takes, but often I am so busy catching a new morsel or idea, I do not spend enough time digesting the last three I started." ~ Miranda

By consciously choosing to take actions that keep you in your center, you will become a clear and precise channel, which will enable you to envision the life you dream for yourself. As you recall, energy follows thought, therefore by having clear intent thoughts, your heart's desires can manifest.

SIMPLE STEPS TO MANIFESTING:

◈ **Be conscious to set intentions in relation to the day ahead.**
This will include meetings, chores or accomplishments that need attention.

◈ **It is also important to set intentions surrounding the bigger picture and the bird's eye view of your life.**
It is so easy to become engulfed in the nitty-gritty of the daily grind that you can forget the point of the journey here on earth is to actually enjoy yourself.

◈ **See what qualities in your life are either being ignored or are missing.**
It may be that you already embody being a brilliant mother, businesswoman, homemaker or artist, yet the quality of being playful, sensual, care free and joyful somehow seems far off in the horizon.

◈ **Setting an intention to invite in whatever quality is void, allows this precious attribute to take a step towards you and meet you in more spontaneous and unexpected ways.**

◈ **Gratitude, gratitude, gratitude always invites in more blessings.**

Rather like the warning on a cigarette packet, remember if a part of your behavior and patterning is to play the victim, be negative or self-defeating, these thoughts and energies may also chase you down. The antidote here is to support yourself with loving acts, live by 'The Foundational Trinity' and take exquisite care of yourself. It is then hard to remain in the mode of 'the cup is half empty'. Be attentive to the state of your mind and emotions, remembering the expression:

"Be careful what you ask for, as you just might get it."

CHOOSE TO FURNISH YOUR MIND

Are you living through the stains from past experiences
or are you choosing to furnish your mind with beliefs
and habits that are authentic to whom you really are
and your values today?

Every experience leaves a footprint. Over time, if the same footprint is trodden repeatedly, the imprint becomes trampled, bruised and even more imbedded in your psyche. Unfortunately, in this scenario, a completely innocent situation could arise. Yet because you are stuck in the old wound, by default the person or situation becomes a reenactment of the past. When this occurs, the unlucky person who has triggered your past conflict ends up in the line of fire and unfortunately becomes target practice for your past anger and unresolved issues.

Imagine you are invited to a very fancy ball. It will be full of fascinating people, delectable food and music to which you can really move. All excited you go to your closet to get out your ball gown and in this scenario, yes, you do own a ball gown! You hold up your beautiful dress and crestfallen you notice a huge stain down the front. Suddenly it all comes flooding back to you. The last ball you attended did not go so well. A little too much red wine mixed with your ex flirting like a Greek God, you scream like a banshee and end up with your head down the toilet throwing up.

THE QUESTION IS WHAT DO YOU DO NOW?

◆ Do you go to the ball in your stained dress, which will be a constant reminder of that pain and humiliation of the past?

◆ Or do you choose to buy a new dress, with no past imprint or stains and go to the ball open to new possibilities and beginnings?

What is being offered here is for you to delve into your closet (your subconscious) and see what old clothes are torn, are stained or no longer fit (bringing your wounds and old hurts to the surface). Then you can choose to release them to 'goodwill' (forgiveness is the key here) so you can then dress yourself in a completely new wardrobe of truth, authenticity, joy, passion and beauty. These expressions of self-love would really be a wonderful choice of fabric here.

The ramblings of the mind do become who you are. Therefore, the next time you are on an internal rant of judgment, bitchiness or condemnation, especially about yourself, pause to turn down the volume and tune back into a more loving dialogue.

WHAT ARE THE FURNISHINGS OF YOUR MIND?

◈ Are they old, tired and worn out?

◈ Are they secondhand from your parents?

◈ Are they judgmental and critical?

◈ Are they stained with past experiences?

◈ Are they loving to you and others?

◈ Are they aligned with your taste and what brings you joy?

◈ Are you living by your truth and making authentic choices?

◈ Is your life ultimately furnished the way you desire?

This analogy can certainly be translated into your physical home, car and environment, as these are literal translations of how you are living in your head.

◊ If your house is in chaos, the chances are you mind is too.

◊ If your car is breaking down, how is your health?

◊ If your paperwork or money is in chaos, how are your stress levels?

Each time you become still, quiet and centered, a new steppingstone is laid. Each time you meditate, pray or go inward, these steppingstones are walked upon and a new pathway is formed. This journey to the self is an internal one and its very existence will cleanse and purify the stains on the mind and the tears of the heart.

*spiritual practices are magnificent
and potent ways to cleanse and purify the mind.*

THE PITFALLS OF SPIRITUALITY

Spiritual bypass leaves the wisdom of the body behind.

Even with all this encouragement and profound reasoning for living a spiritual life, there is still a word of warning. If you are not grounded in your body and taking care of your "Foundational Trinity" through sleep, nourishing food and exercise, it does not matter how hard you pray or meditate. The physical form will give up if ignored.

Imagine you were building a magnificent temple or church. In all its glory, its steeples would reach the heavens, the colored glass would reflect the light, and the mosaic floors would inspire devotion, yet there was no money to build a strong foundation. All the attention went to the higher realms. Eventually your beautiful sacred house would fall.

"I have a friend who was a dedicated Buddhist for many years. During his spiritual practice, he would sit cross-legged for hours. Now he has pain in both knees which limits his ability to sit in meditation and ski, his other love." ~ Miranda

It really is all about balancing your human and spiritual beings. Both need to be cherished, honored and obeyed. If one aspect is eclipsing the other, then it may be time to shift and rebalance. If one expression is non-existent then it is definitely time to devote some attention to this beleaguered and ignored self.

"In my own life I study with my spiritual teacher twice a year. One year, due to buying a house, I foolishly decided not to visit. I paid dearly, not financially but emotionally and spiritually. By spending five precious days in his presence, I received the teachings I love and I fill my well to overflowing. It seems that this infusion lasts about six months. I certainly take sips and nibbles along the way in my mundane life, but my feast is the immersion of my spirit, into this world for that precious pocket of time." ~ Miranda

There is always a danger if you bypass the body to reach spiritual relief before you are ready. It is in the wisdom of the body that many emotions, reactions and humanities are held. When these are deemed too painful or too much to handle it can be tempting to disassociate from the physical form, instead of actually dropping inward to listen to her profound message. If these human responses are ignored too long, they are then left to fester in the cells of the body completely unattended to.

By choosing to be present to the emptiness, pain or grief of being human, the emotion are then lived through and processed. Then when appropriate you will naturally transcend to the higher levels of forgiveness and love. It is also important to pay attention if you are not speaking your truth and honoring that you are a physical, mental, emotional and spiritual being. Sometimes being overly spiritual can lead to being taken advantage of.

'Loving kindness' can become 'she is a push over' if it is not connected and grounded to a strong sense of self and some backbone. Saying no can sometimes be the hardest act of all. Yet in many scenarios, it is the absolute right action of love.

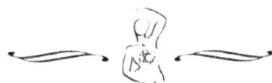

Remember, loving kindness to the self
is always the ultimate and most grace-filled of spiritual practices
and is available in every moment of every day.
~ Anonymous

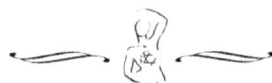

THE ART OF PLACEMENT

The Nine Palaces.

To remain healthy and balanced it is vital to keep a continuous stream of positive energy flowing throughout your mind, body and spirit. It is also imperative for your well-being to align this flow of energy in your living space and home.

Fortunately, there are ancient traditions, which can guide you in this art form. One practice is Vastu Shastra, the Vedic science of architecture and design of temples, homes and buildings. What yoga is for the body, Vatsu is for the physical environments facilitating health, harmony and balance. Often referred to as 'Indian Feng Shui ', Vastu actually pre-dates the Chinese tradition of Feng Shui. Similarly, Feng Shui is like acupuncture for your home.

Instead of points in the body being stimulated, the spaces in the house are energized to release blockages and to restore a healthy and vital flow. In either method, bringing change to your surroundings will transform the energy and flow.

The customs and teachings of Feng Shui incorporates the physical elements and objects in your living or workspace and uses them as a way to move stagnant energy, clear blockages and strengthen your beneficial intentions. It is all about the placement of certain objects in order to enhance the 'Chi', energy or Pranic flow.

Each area of a space correlates to a specific aspect of your life such as love, health or career. By enhancing each quadrant, the qualities within them will be harmonized.

By consciously choosing to improve a certain area, such as the prosperity quadrant for example, you are opening the channels, clearing out the residue and creating a space for abundance, wealth and riches to flourish in your life.

FENG SHUI CONCEPTS ARE RELATIVELY SIMPLE:

◆ Your home, office, car, desk or any building is divided into nine equal quadrants. Think of a Rubik's Cube.

◆ Each of the nine quadrants or Palaces has a specific purpose.

◆ Certain numbers, colors, objects, shapes and intentions strengthen the area.

◆ Clutter, mess, trash, broken items, dust and dirt and ignoring the area will limit and dishevel the energy

It is fascinating how you can be having an issue in your life and you then check out the correlating space in your home. Often it will be in disarray or chaos.

"I had a client who was having an influx of health and family issues. I asked her what was going on in this area of her house and she revealed that it was being used as a rather messy construction site to redo a bathroom upstairs. Both areas of health and family were being pulled apart and not being treated with respect. I asked her to speak with her contractor about cleaning up his mess that was possibly causing her ill health. This was accomplished and her medical tests came back perfectly fine."
~ Miranda

BASIC GUIDELINES TO FENG SHUI YOUR LIFE:

◆ **Feng Shui is all about energy.**
Therefore, do not get too rigid if it is unclear whether a specific area is in a certain quadrant or another. Rather like a rainbow, the quadrants merge and overlap. It is all about intention.

◆ **Any building, room or desk is divided into nine equal quadrants.**
Imagine you have a bird's eye view.

◆ **The doorway into the space translates as the entrance.**
The nine quadrants then sit behind the doorway. It does not matter if the door is centered, to the right or left.

◆ **If the space or object is not square or apiece is missing, the empty space needs to be counted as the whole, even if it is in the garden.**
Imagine extending the lines along the walls into the missing area. The point where these two imaginary lines meet is an area to enhance, such as placing a plant, a tree or hanging a wind chime or crystal. Also, pay attention to enhancing items elsewhere that correlate to the missing quadrant.

◆ **You can divide any space such as your garage into the nine quadrants.**

◆ **You can also divide a separate room, closet, drawer, garden shed or your car.**

◆ **If a quadrant is missing, it is vital to enhance the missing Palace.**
For example if your prosperity corner is missing, you would want to enhance the prosperity corner in all the other rooms of the house. This would mean adding some gold coins, amethyst, a money plant or some valuable possessions. You can follow the walls of the house and see where the two lines meet in the missing quadrant. Here, you can hang a faceted crystal, a wind chime, plant a tree or bury a crystal correlated to the area.

◆ **Separate buildings that are not attached have their own nine Palaces.**
Examples of these are garages, garden sheds and guesthouses.

◆ **Clearing clutter, old unwanted junk, broken objects or items you do not care for, is a huge energy enhancer.**
It may help closing the door to the chaotic closet or garage because what the eye does not see, the heart does not grieve, or so they say. Yet in the world of energy, that disorganized drawer is still draining, blocking and wasting valuable energy.

◈ **Sometimes, an area can be configured to enhance two Palaces at once.**
A room may be in the love and relationship area of the house's Feng Shui quadrant, yet when dividing the room into nine areas, you will also want to develop all the other eight aspects. This means that along with many pairs of hearts in the space, you will also want to add crystals into the career area for example and some gold coins into the prosperity corner.

◈ **In the love and relationship corner, pair objects so there are always two.**
This will enhance partnership. Do not have a single mirror hanging at the foot of the bed. It may invite in a third party!

◈ **Use the associated number, color, shape, or element to enhance a quadrant.**
An example is a red candle that you light in the fame and reputation Palace or eight shiny pennies or gold dollars in the wealth and prosperity corner. By using the color and shape associated to the Palace.

◈ **If a certain corner or area seems unwelcoming, dark or stagnant, you can hang around a faceted glass crystal, a wind chime or place a lamp.**
This will enhance the flow to the area and re-introduce chi and energy.

◈ **Poison arrows are another energy block.**
This is when a corner of a table, furniture or wall is pointing at you while you are spending time in bed, on a sofa or at your desk. Next time you are in one of these places, look around and see if any corners are directly aimed at you. Remedy this by hanging a faceted crystal just in front of the poison arrow.

◈ **Be inventive and creative. There is no right or wrong here.**
This is all about bringing in your version, taste and energy to enhance each quadrant. For example in the Family Palace where you want to bring in the element of wood, you could use a wooden picture frame, a piece of driftwood, a wooden bench or a string of wooden beads.

◆ Always pay attention if an area of your life is not working and check out the corresponding area in your living space.
Then clean up the area, clear it out and add in the beneficial Feng Shui elements to bring happiness and harmony back into your life.

◆ Also, if an area of your house is falling apart, do something!
See what area it corresponds to and fix it up.

◆ For information on how to Feng Shui your living or work spaces, please refer to 'The Nine Palaces' chart.
This will give you a guide for you to fulfill all aspects and corners of your life.

Being conscious of your home and your living environment will change your life.

"I was having some money flow issues, so I decided to go around and enhance the prosperity corners of my home. I used eight red and gold Chinese fortune envelopes, placed a gold dollar coin in each one and discretely and placed them in each of the wealth corners. The next day I found an envelope with one thousand dollars cash on my kitchen table. A generous friend had left it as a gift. And a gift it certainly was."
~ Miranda

You can download a copy of 'The Nine Palaces' chart
from Miranda's website at:
www.MirandaJBarrett.com/product/the-nine-palaces-of-feng-shui

THE STILL LAKE OF THE MIND

That which is purest in me has never uttered a word.

Spirituality can bring forth a whole new level of consciousness. The use of spiritual practice will support and invite you to become silent and travel inward, receiving peace of mind and a glimpse of who you truly are.

The aspect that is recognized through stillness can be called the witness or even the watcher within. This observer knows you are not just a mind and a body. This facet of you is pure energy from source. It is unemotional, unattached and infinite. It is what remains when all else dies or fades away. It is what never changes among all that transforms. It is not dependent on this life or your survival, as it is always part of the whole.

In the following meditation, instead of connecting to the distorted facade of human emotions and restrictions, you will drop into the expanse of stillness of just being. From this perspective, all is possible. There are no limitations, deaths or denials.

◆ Take a few deep relaxing breaths.

◆ Imagine yourself dropping down into the silent depths of a lake.
All is quiet and motionless. As you sit deep below the surface of your life, connect to the part of you that is infinite and unchanged. Invite in the witness who will allow you to be the observer of all that is happening around you.

◆ Enjoy how quiet and peaceful it is in the depths of your being.

◆ Imagine the surface of the lake with turbulence, commotion and people.
The waves break the rays of light with shadow. There on the surface, life is happening in all its hubbub and activity, good and bad.

◆ **There is a tendency to attach to the activity above.**
The intention is to keep a connection to the still waters. Do not judge the yearning to connect to the outside world. Just observe and witness the inclination and gently bring yourself back.

◆ **Keep your connection to the watcher within and continue to drop yourself deeper into the stillness.**

◆ **When a storm comes, keep your anchor in the tranquil waters.**
From this place of stability, you will not be easily disturbed from your center.

As you nourish your connection to the observer,
you will always weather the storm by aligning with unchanging,
infinite awareness of who you truly are.

SPIRITUAL CLEANSING

You may not be able to control your first thought
as is catapults into your head,
but you can control every thought thereafter.

As a human being, you may choose to clean out a closet, your car or even your body because the chaos and dysfunction becomes loud enough that it can no longer be ignored. This is particularly true with the body as physical pain is a constant reminder to take action.

"I am always amazed when I give myself a day to spring clean, how good I feel afterwards, even if I am filthy and tired." ~ Miranda

Yet what about cleaning out the mind, the thoughts and the emotions? If only it was that easy to throw out an old box of betrayal or to give away bags of self-loathing. As the saying goes:

One woman's trash is another woman's treasure.

Under the premise that your outside world begins with your internal thoughts, it begs the question why more time, money and energy is not spent on cleaning out the cesspool of the mind and thoughts. It seems like such a stellar investment. Yet in reality it appears as though much more energy is devoted to the externally manifested world, rather than fine-tuning the internal workings of the psyche.

Here is some spiritual food for thought.

A SPIRITUAL PURIFICATION:

◆ The next time you decide to clean, ponder the idea of starting with your mind.

◆ Choose to live a day with only loving thoughts for yourself.

◈ Each time an unkind or critical thought pops in, and they will, choose not to follow that path of loathing and self-destruct.
In the beginning, this will be all about disciplining the mind, rather like a badly behaved puppy. 'No, you will not chew my favorite shoes.'

◈ Instead, choose a loving thought for yourself.
Counteract the meanness with love. Create an antidote for the illness of self-hatred with the remedy of kindness.

◈ Treat yourself internally as you would someone you dearly love.

◈ This practice can also be used for judgmental thoughts towards another.

It is all very well thinking that harsh, critical tirades in your head do not matter because no one else hears them. Wrong. You hear them and you feel them. The thought then becomes energy and the energy travels throughout your body, is stored in your cells, and eventually becomes your physically manifested reality.

"After years of meditating, I now realize that it does not matter if my mind is on a rampage of trailing delinquency, as long as I remember I am not my mind and keep drawing back to my center and core of who I am. This is what I strengthen each time I choose to travel inward. I am literally spiritually spring-cleaning the cobwebs, dust and droppings of my rambling psyche." ~ Miranda

POSSIBLE SPIRITUAL CLEANING:

The following are some beliefs, tapes and mental thoughts and habits that might well be cluttering your mind and therefore your world. By cleansing these thoughts, you will ultimately become lighter, freer, emptier and more willing and able to see new views and beliefs: ones that support, nourish and help manifest the world of your dreams.

CULPRITS YOU RESONATE WITH AND REPEAT OFTEN:

◊ Thinking you need to be right

◊ I am too fat, thin, old, wrinkly...

◊ Comparing yourself to others

◊ Phobias and obsessions

◊ Fear to speak up or act or not being enough

◊ The belief you are alone and unsupported

◊ The belief you have to do it all yourself

◊ Judgments and regrets

◊ Fear of looking foolish or the times you screwed up

◊ The cup is always half empty

◊ Insecurities and paranoia

◊ Fearing the outcome before you know it

◊ Believing you need to please everyone

◊ Caring if people like you

◊ Anger and resentments

◊ Jealousy, envious and vengeful thoughts

◊ (Fill in your own here!)

chose to diminish their significance.

THREE CUPS FULL

How are your cups? Are they half-full, half-empty or so full of crud that you cannot see the water?

Just so you know, this is not referring to breast size! This is about taking a good long look at your life as the observer and becoming aware of the state of your world.

◆ **Visualize a cup of water in front of you.**
  At first glance, it looks like a perfectly innocent glass of water. Yet upon closer inspection you notice sediment or dirt on the bottom.

◆ **Now imagine you take a spoon and start to stir up the water in the glass.**
  All of a sudden, there is no clarity or clear water. It is all mucked up with the dirt. In fact, you cannot even see through the glass anymore.

◆ **Then you let it settle.**
  It takes time but eventually the sediment drops to the bottom. Yet each time there is commotion, up it stirs again.

◆ **Now you decide to take another glass and pour the clear settled water from the original water glass into the new one.**
  A little bit of the sediment is transferred but not much. Again, you let it settle.

◆ **Eventually you decide to get a brand new glass and fill it with fresh water and pour the dirty water down the drain where it belongs.**

◆ **Later you notice a fly has landed in your new glass...**
  This may have felt a little bit like an experiment, but hopefully you get the gist.

Life is a continuous journey of clarity and collecting dirt. Sometimes you get to stir the pot, other times life does the stirring. The importance here is to know that life can be dirty. Periodically, empty the containers of the past, spring-cleaning and knowing to start afresh is always priceless.

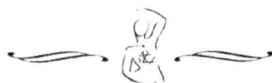

"May not one take muddy water
and make it clear by keeping still?"
~ Lao Tzu

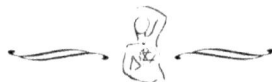

WHAT FEEDS YOU?

Nourishing and nurturing your spirit.

Connecting to your higher self is a very personal and individual journey and only you will know when you have arrived. The joy is everyone has the opportunity and the gift of exploring and going on this quest. Do not neglect your soul or deprive it of nourishment.

"Being near the ocean or on top of a mountain is where I seem to find one of my versions of God. It is as though the world stands still in all its glory and I am acutely aware of the present moment. The vast wonder and merciless wisdom and fury of mother earth comes alive in me. In fact, when I go for too long without the sea, I start to long and pine for her. Rather like my dear friend, the other Miranda who also nourishes my being." ~ Miranda

Take a moment to ponder and write down what feeds your spiritual being.

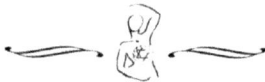

*"Knock, And He'll open the door
Vanish, And He'll make you shine like the sun
Fall, And He'll raise you to the heavens
Become nothing, And He'll turn you into everything"*

~ Rumi

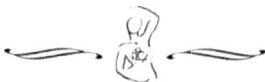

A DAILY SPIRITUAL PRACTICE
One day at a time.

This is an invitation to embody higher spiritual aspects on a daily basis. Each day a new word and spiritual consciousness is chosen and lived by.

Let us say you choose to embody the word love.

How this translates is that throughout the next twenty-four hours you will set the intention to come from a place of love, no matter what the situation! This will include love for others, for animals, for strangers, for nature, for your computer and most importantly for yourself.

The following words are offerings and suggestions. You may follow them exactly in order or choose the one that calls to you that day. You can also determine your own personal quality that resonates with you. It is helpful to write the word out somewhere you will see it or with lipstick on a mirror to remind yourself of your spiritual nature.

◆ **Abundance**
  Live in the overflowing fullness and wealth of all you have already received. Be open to receiving the riches surrounding you and be grateful for the blessings bestowed upon your life.

◆ **Adventure**
  Soften all your edges and lean into whatever is present for you right now. Sanction what is and give yourself permission to let go of resistance and just be.

◆ **Allow**
  Awaken to the spirit of adventure, which may be lying dormant within you. Enliven and excite yourself. Take a chance to venture out into the world of the unknown.

◈ Ask

Acknowledge what you need. Inquire into what you truly seek. Allow vulnerability by asking for help and support. Know if you do not ask, the answer is already a no. Become curious of another by asking what they might need.

◈ Beauty

Beauty is in the eye of the beholder. Become the one who is awe inspired by your own beauty and grace. Remember, true beauty is not only captured by the eyes, but is also felt in the heart.

◈ Breathe

Deepen your breath. With each, invite more inspiration and expiration of life force into your being. As you inhale, receive. As you exhale, release and let go.

◈ Centered

Remain authentic to your true self. Stay well balanced as you consciously stand in your integrity, no matter whom or what comes your way.

◈ Change

Remember, change is the only constant. Welcome the transformation of outmoded beliefs and habits into new ways of being.

◈ Commitment

Release all feelings of obligation and commit whole-heartedly to yourself. When you uphold your promise to honor this commitment, trust is built, as you naturally become your own best friend and mentor.

◈ Communication

Be honest with yourself and all who cross your path. Exchange thoughts and ideas that convey your authentic self. Be conscious to listen to others as a way to create shared understanding, even if you disagree.

◆ Compassion
Allow yourself to be present to the powerfully deep awareness of another's suffering. Acknowledge the desire to alleviate the distress, yet choose to be present to the feeling. Do so without actually taking action or attempting to solve the situation.

◆ Confidence
Walk tall in your power. Remember all of who you are. Believe in your own worth and beauty. Acknowledge all the gifts, talents and extraordinary abilities that already lie within you.

◆ Consciousness
Knowingly activate your mind and senses as you awaken to your life. Become fully aware of the miraculous world surrounding you. Wake up to this present moment. It is all there truly is.

◆ Counsel
Open up to the guidance and inner wisdom of your own intuition and counsel. Remember this inner voice may whisper its teachings. Become still enough to listen and then respond accordingly.

◆ Courage
True courage comes from the strength within the heart. Fill yourself with love and valor to become the one for whom to die. This bravery will help keep you aligned to your authentic values even in the face of judgment or criticism.

◆ Creativity
Play in the dance of creation itself and manifest your dreams, visions and ideas into existence. Follow your inspiration and design a life worth living.

◆ Dignity
Never require yourself to sacrifice your dignity, integrity or self worth. Lay the grace of this noble quality on the altar of your life as you honor yourself and others with deep love, appreciation and respect. Know you are worthy of a richly dignified life.

◆ **Discipline**
Let go of the concept of rules and regulations. Replace the harshness of judgment with love. Invoke a strong alignment with what you know to be true. Use self-discipline as a loving way to remain authentic to yourself.

◆ **Empower**
Endow yourself with your own sovereignty to become the wholehearted authority of your life. Then claim the neutral nature of power to fuel your own capacity and sustain this journey with virtue and the sanction of grace.

◆ **Emptiness**
Empty your mind and being of all future desires and wishes. Be present to the power and vastness of the moment. Stop doing and just be. Drop into the void.

◆ **Faith**
Faith and fear cannot occupy the same space. Nurture faith in yourself and your choices. Let go of fear and become loyal to your own sense of knowing.

◆ **Flexibility**
Become like the ebb and flow of water. Let go of controlling, planning and having it your way. Surrender your agendas and expectations. As you relinquish control, there is no longer a need for pressure to charter your course.

◆ **Forgiveness**
Renounce any feelings of anger and resentment. Release your desire for revenge and punishment. Have mercy on yourself and others, allowing love to fill your heart instead. Forgive yourself for being fallible and human.

◆ **Freedom**
Liberate yourself from the shackles of fear. Invoke the freedom to determine your actions without the restriction of limiting beliefs. Abandon all restraints and deliver your life into the hands of ease and grace. Remember, freedom is not worth having if you do not have the freedom to make a mistake.

◆ Generosity
Willingly give from the overflow of your time, money, energy and love. Bestow without any expectation of return reward. In this pure giving, you will also receive.

◆ Give
When giving, bestow directly from your heart. Award another with a loving and kind gesture of support. Yet always discern if you have the gift to give without resentment. If not, give to yourself first.

◆ Grace
Live your day in simple elegance with the free and unmerited favor of the divine essence of grace. Allow elegance to adorn your existence and dignify your worth.

◆ Gratitude
Gratitude is the most fertile of all soils in which to plant intentions. Continually express your deep sense of thankfulness for all.

◆ Harmony
Free yourself from conflict and expectations. Align with the melodies and rhythms of the universe. Relax into a balanced relationship with existence.

◆ Humility
Exalt within the simplicity of being humble and of this earth. Live greatly as you release the artificial nature of pride. Allow the essence of gentle respect and not knowing lead the way as arrogance and fear melt in the presence of humility.

◆ Innocence
Return to innocence. For a precious moment in time, release being responsible or a grownup. Devote yourself to the pure simplicity that you were before knowledge and experience stained your life. Delight in the wonder of your childlike nature.

◆ Integrity

Align with the purity of your own being. Become intimate with what you know to be true and what you aspire to and deeply value. Be sincere in the virtue of living within your own honor.

◆ Intention

Setting clear and meaningful goals helps you to align with your purpose. Make a wish for your day and intend for this dream to come true.

◆ Intuition

Listen to the keen insights and wisdom of your inner perceptions and instincts. Know this inner guidance will always love, support, and show you the way.

◆ Joy

Rejoice and spend precious moments encompassing the essence of pleasure, revelry and delight. Spontaneously celebrate in the festivities of life.

◆ Kindness

Become open to your own tenderness and loving ways. Receive the benevolence of kindheartedness from yourself and others. Once your heart is full of gentle kindness, generously give this gift to those who cross your path.

◆ Laughter

Always have a sense of humor about yourself before anyone else gets a chance. Remember, laughter is a free medicine and a powerful healer.

◆ Love

Release all that is not love and choose to express loving heartfelt acts. Immerse in the selfless affection, tenderness and concern you feel for yourself and another.

◆ Mystery

Calm your sweet mind and drop into Divine knowledge where the paradox and the unexplained nature of life is revealed in the glory of not knowing. Receive comfort from the wise yet simple truths of what cannot be defined.

◆ **Passion**
Stir the desire to awaken fervor and passion in your life. Call upon that which is so powerful and compelling, it will eclipse all logic and restraint. Rejoice in the delight and adoration of this life force.

◆ **Patience**
Willingly and lovingly accept, tolerate and embrace the obstacles in your day with calmness and grace. You never know the unforeseen reason for the delay.

◆ **Pay it forward**
If you have plenty, give your wealth, if you only have a little, you can always give from your heart. In the giving, you will also receive.

◆ **Peace**
Reconcile internal conflicts with yourself by simply meeting all fractions with love, compassion and respect. No longer oppose what is. Peace is born of understanding, therefore restore unity and surrender to the heartfelt direction, which invokes a sense of harmony and ease.

◆ **Play**
Allow your childlike wonder to come out and play. Let go of being responsible. Laugh for no reason, dance with abandon and play just because you can. Revel in lightheartedness and have no other agenda but to have fun.

◆ **Purity**
Cleanse your thoughts from all that limits, harms and pollutes you. This will set you free. Embody self-love as the doorway into to cleansing the movements of the mind and allow your actions to become pure in mind, body and spirit.

◆ **Purpose**
Live your life on purpose. Aspire to make deliberate and conscious decisions and actions, which support your goal of living a full and authentic life.

◆ **Radiance**
Radiate and share the bright shining light that dwells within you. Garner your light and allow whom you truly are to shine by taking exquisite care of yourself.

◆ **Receiving**
Pause the momentum of your life and become present to receive all the gifts already waiting for you. Gratitude will open your heart to accept the blessings.

◆ **Rejuvenation**
Give yourself the gift of luxurious self-care. This will allow you to recharge and restore your well-being. Allow this to refill you to overflowing.

◆ **Respect**
Know that respect and trust is earned. Hold and instill within yourself such high regard that others will respond with a deep sense of reverence and admiration.

◆ **Reverence**
Become one whose presence alone imbues a feeling of trust and reverence. As you hold yourself in high regard and respect, you will recognize these qualities in others. Devote yourself to that which fills you with awe.

◆ **Serenity**
Peace is not determined by the state of the outside world, but is the precious ability to remain tranquil and calm amid the chaos of the storm. As you observe the turmoil rather than react, the space for serenity is born.

◆ **Silence**
Revel in the strength and power of silence. Quiet your mind and senses. Choose not to speak unless what you have to say will improve upon the silence.

◆ **Simplicity**
Allow the qualities of grace and ease to flow through your life. Draw your attention to all that naturally embodies purity and innocence. Release having to adorn and complicate that which is already filled with beauty.

◆ **Sovereignty**
Reign in the supreme and unrestricted power of your own autonomy. Liberate yourself from limiting beliefs. Inspire your own freedom to choose, act and behave in rich alignment with who you know yourself to be.

◆ **Spontaneity**

Be willing to let go of tightly holding the reins of life. Release your grip, be open and allow the wild forces of spontaneity and freedom to arise from within you. Awaken to your natural impulse and internal callings.

◆ **Stillness**

Surrender to not doing. Allow the tranquility and peace of being still fulfill and guide you into right action. As you sit in your still point, all possibilities will be revealed and the way forward will become known.

◆ **Surrender**

Yield and give yourself up to the ebb and flow of life, regardless of which direction it may take you. True surrender takes courage from the heart and releases all expectations, agendas and outcomes.

◆ **Symbolism**

Be open to the metaphors and symbols that are all around you and enrich the tapestry of life. They may be a whisper or a shout, a tiny glimpse or a blinding stare. Yet the secret is to pay attention, listen to the message and to act upon your internal wisdom.

◆ **Synchronicity**

Choose to let go of your limiting beliefs so you can invite in the spontaneous and meaningful coincidences that life affords. As you align with the forces of nature, indulge in the guidance these parallel encounters can provide for you.

◆ **Tenderness**

Yield to the soft and delicate touch of being sensitive. Immerse yourself in the delicate vulnerability of a tender heart. Have mercy on yourself and allow this fragility to awaken, knowing you always have a warrior's strength within you.

◆ **Transformation**

Relinquish the old ways that no longer serve you. Partner courage with surrender and allow them to guide you on this life journey of transformation and change. As these beliefs are reduced to ash, surrender to the void of not knowing. Yet, have faith that the metamorphosis of new life is beginning.

◆ **Truth**

Live honestly with honor, strength, integrity and love. Choose to eliminate dishonesty in your life by speaking your truth and saying no when appropriate.

◆ **Willingness**

Be open to confront the uncomfortable and the illusions in your life. Relinquish your attachment to empty agendas and any resistance to positive change. Be willing to take chances, to make mistakes and even to fail. Cheerfully consent to what you know to be true. Be willing, ready and able to choose an authentic life.

◆ **Wonder**

Fill yourself with admiration and amazement at this mystery called life as you return to the innocence of awe. Marvel and allow surprise and curiosity to lead your way and remember how wisdom begins with wonder.

"On a day where I chose to live by the quality of "receiving", many wonderful and unexpected gifts came my way. The 'Piece de la Resistance' was when I had my head in the fishpond trying to fix the filter and a friend turned up unexpectedly, helped me with the problem and also gave me a dozen fresh eggs from his chickens. On the next day, I chose communication and by six in the evening I had had so much dialogue with so many people that I turned the phone off." ~ Miranda

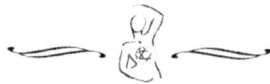

"when looking up the definition of emptiness on line, the screen literally showed up blank. Need I say more?"
~ Miranda

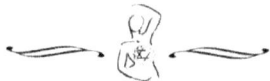

REVEAL MORE TRUTH

"This is my simple religion. There is no need for temples;
no need for complicated philosophy.
Our own brain, our own heart is our temple;
the philosophy is kindness."
~ Dali Lama

Your vocation for the next few weeks is an internal journey to invoke your spiritual essence. By choosing to live a spiritual life, you will naturally fill your well to overflowing, saying nothing of the gift you will be giving to those who surround you. It can be a wonderful life when you embody spirituality in unison with your physicality.

◈ Spend some time reading your guidebook.
   By consciously connecting to spiritual writings is a spiritual practice.

◈ Enjoy making any moment a spiritual moment.

◈ If you have a situation or person who is bothering you or you are still mad at them, write a 'Letter of Truth' and burn it.

◈ If the Feng Shui tickled your fancy, you can spend a few minutes a day creatively rearranging the energy of your home.

◈ Choose to feast daily on your connection to spirituality.

◈ For some of you, setting up an altar or a sacred space in your home could be an auspicious spiritual awakening.

◈ And saving the best till last, enjoy 'A Daily Spiritual Practice'.

You can order a copy of Miranda's 'Inspiration Cards'

from her website at:

www.MirandaJBarrett.com/product/inspiration-cards

Love and blessings to you on this sacred journey back to the Self,

Miranda

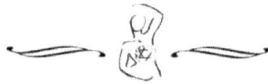

"There is a candle in your heart,
ready to be kindled. There is a void in your soul,
ready to be filled. You feel it, don't you?"

~ Rumi

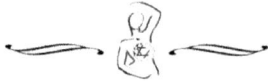

SPIRITUAL AWAKENING

when the red thread of human desire becomes unbearable.

Yearn
Say yes
Scream no

Pray
Meditate
Be still

Retreat
Study
Seek wisdom, knowledge and answers

Purify
Transform
Initiate

Evolve
Expand
Becoming enlightened

Such light
Such consciousness

Too awake
Too bright
Retreat to the witness

Separate
Unattached
Observing from the ethers

Feels dull
Too dry
A longing to dance with spirit

Such joy
Undying bliss
Rich lavish adornments of God

The feast of devotion awakened

Grace
Echelon
Agapae

To experience all as the infinite
You, me, the stranger
You, me, the torrid
You, me, the radiant

All still human
Yet always infinite

Let the dance within begin
Falling back into the arms of infinite potential
Awakening to the divine emptiness

ABOUT MIRANDA

A spirited guide and mentor.

Miranda is a passionate and devoted leader. Her loving and wise support will guide you on a transformational journey as her powerful teachings unveil the truth of who you are. Her gift is to offer potent tools, which inspire exquisite and beautiful self-care and empower you to live the fullest and most authentic life possible. As a mentor and guide, Miranda deeply walks her talk and is fearless about her own path of self-discovery, as she weaves the sacred into the mundane.

The simple, yet powerful premise offered by the mystic Rumi is the foundation of Miranda's philosophy and mission:

> *"Never give from the depths of your well,*
> *always give from your overflow."*

Miranda gives Council and Guidance for the Mind, Body and Spirit. With a background in Nutrition and Energy work, Miranda is the Creator of 'A Woman's Truth' and 'The Spirit of Energy', an Author, a Workshop and Retreat Leader, a Reiki Master and Yoga and Meditation teacher. Miranda studies under the guidance of her Beloved teachers Rod Stryker and Adyashanti.

To speak with or follow Miranda, please call or visit:

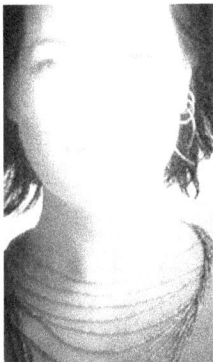

Phone: 626~798~6544
eMail: Info@MirandaJBarrett.com
Website: www.MirandaJBarrett.com
Facebook: Miranda J Barrett
Twitter: MirandaJBarrett

ABOUT HELENA

A visionary artist.

Helena Nelson-Reed is a visionary artist whose primary medium is watercolor. Born in Seattle, Washington, she was raised in Marin County and Napa Valley, California and today lives in Illinois. A largely self-taught artist whose educational emphasis and degree is in psychology, Nelson-Reed's primary focus is exploring the collective consciousness and the portrayal of archetypal imagery in the tradition of Carl Jung and Joseph Campbell. Rendered in luminous watercolor technique often described as ephemeral, Nelson-Reed's paintings are created in extraordinary detail, pushing the medium of watercolor past the usual limits. Her work may be found in private collections, book covers, magazines and cd covers. Nelson-Reed also has a line of jewelry, calendars and greeting cards.

Helena's Mission:

My images can be interpreted many ways, and for some will serve as portal to the mythic landscape. Descriptions providing background about each painting are available by request. Navigating and translating myth into contemporary wisdom is the traditional way of transmitting information though a shamanic and multi-cultural practice.

Myth, fairy, folk and spiritual lore describe divine beings and supernatural life forms arriving unbidden and disguised. In our earthly dimension, mortals often play similar roles in the lives of one another. Destinies and energies collide and interact, visible and invisible forces are at work. The mythic realms are timeless, offering insight and inspiration. While my paintings have a positive energy, many have roots in the shadows of life experience and human psyche; like the lotus blossom rooted in pond mud. For many, life is one challenge followed by the next, like beads on an endless string.

Take heart! Like goddess Inanna, one may navigate the underworld, move through dark places yet return to the realms of light battle scarred but wiser, richer for the experience. Read the ancient tales, the great mythic literature; draw strength, for they are repositories of wisdom.

Visit Helena's website for her art, purchase information and art to wear jewelry:

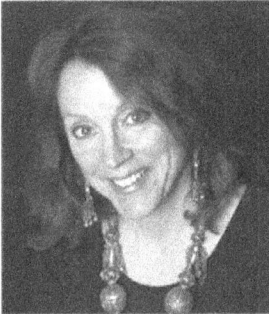

eMail: HNelsonReed@Gmail.com

Websites: www.HelenaNelsonReed.com

www.etsy.com/shop/HelenaNelsonReed

Blog: www.dancingdovestudio.blogspot.com

Facebook: MorningDove Design By Helena

MIRANDA'S WORLD

*Ways to stay connected
and aligned with your truth.*

BOOKS:

A Woman's Truth
A life truly worth living.

Priceless teachings reveal your transformational
journey ahead. Obstacles to self-care are explored
as clear and loving intentions are conceived.

The Grandeur of Sleep
Permission to rest.

Miraculous benefits are realized as the worlds of sleep,
relaxation and rejuvenation are explored and deeply honored.

Nourishing Nutrition
Reclaim your health and vitality.

Reap the bountiful rewards while eating as nature intended.
Claim your health and vitality with these simple,
yet powerful tools to nourish and heal your body.

Embodying Movement
Ground your whole being.

Restore balance in your life. Discover how to embrace
your whole being through the life-enhancing benefits of body movement.

Body Care
Cherish your body as a temple.

Learn to honor your extraordinary body
as a living temple and listen to the healing messages she whispers.

Feminine Power
Fully access your supreme birthright.

Welcome and reclaim this intrinsic privilege while living
in harmonious balance between the masculine and the feminine.

The Abundance Of Wealth
Receive the gifts of prosperity.

Understand the energy flow of prosperity and weave
the threads of abundance throughout the tapestry of your life.

Find Your Authentic Voice

The courage to express who you truly are.

Your greatest ally is born
when you courageously speak your truth and claim your unique power.

Loving Yourself

A Love Affair to the Self.

As you become highly attuned to your own needs,
allow love to lead the way. Grant yourself permission
to honor and express your heart's truest desires.
Love yourself no matter what.

Living A Spiritual Life

Ground your divine essence here on earth.

Discover what spirituality means to you, by consciously
living between the two worlds of the sacred and the mundane.

Service As A Way of Life

Ignite the fire of love to truly be of service.

By utilizing the gems of exquisite self-care
on a daily basis and honoring your truth, your mission of service is born.

The Crowning Glory
Fully Rejoice in Being You.

A celebration overflowing with love,
blessings, grace and gratitude. Stand confident within
your truth as your mind begins to serve your heart.

The Food Of Life
The versatile vegetable.

More than just a cookbook,
a comprehensive guide for nourishing your life.

Reiki
The spirit of Energy.

An insightful guidebook full of wisdom
which introduces you to the potent and healing world of Reiki.

CARDS:

Inspiration Cards
A daily Spiritual Practice.

Sixty-Five cards with simple yet inspirational qualities
to live by and an insightful guidebook to lead the way.

CD'S:

The Grandeur of sleep and Rejuvenating Rest

An ancient healing art of rest and relaxation.

Simple yet profound practices, which alleviate stress and tension allowing your mind, body and spirit to heal, restore and replenish.

TO ORDER PLEASE VISIT:

www.MirandaJBarrett.com
www.Amazon.com

*All books are available in printed or eBook form.

TESTIMONIES

to 'A Woman's Truth' teachings.

"I am forever grateful for the teachings of 'A Woman's Truth' and the loving support of Miranda Barrett as our guide. It has been a journey of uncovering truths about myself that I had long since forgotten, clearing away emotional debris that no longer serves me and taking concrete steps to move into patterns that are deeply loving and caring for myself. I can truly say that miracles are occurring in my life because of my decision to take my self-care into my own hands and radically honor myself. I have a well of love and energy to help those around me that I had forgotten about. Discovering that energy is all about "filling up my well' first, an oxymoron in today's pressured culture, but an ancient truth that is the secret to my happiness. Thank you Miranda for reminding me of my true power, grace and beauty as a woman."

Nicole ~ Nutritionist ~ Altadena, CA

"The journey of 'A Woman's Truth' invites me to intentionally contemplate the inner and outer workings of my life and gives me the courage to transform myself so that I can be more like...myself! Miranda's wisdom and clarity shed light on even the darkest places in life, and her guidance equips me with practical tools to transform my setbacks into self-love and personal victories. I'm grateful beyond words."

Johanna ~ Mother of three ~ Altadena, CA

www.ingramcontent.com/pod-product-compliance
Lightning Source LLC
Chambersburg PA
CBHW081159270326
41930CB00014B/3219